HOW TO MAKE A HOME GYM

A Comprehensive Guide to Building, Equipping, and Using Your Home Gym on a Budget

Curtis Wood

How to make a home gym

Copyright © 2024 by Curtis Wood

All rights reserved.
No part of this work may be reproduced, distributed, or transmitted in any form or by any means, including photocopying, recording, or other electronic or mechanical methods, without the prior written permission of the copyright holder, except in the case of brief quotations embodied in critical reviews and certain other noncommercial uses permitted by copyright law.

How to make a home gym

Table of content

Introduction 4
Chapter 1: Benefits of a Home Gym 8
Chapter 2: Assessing Your Space 13
Chapter 3: Setting Your Budget 19
Chapter 4: Planning Your Home Gym Layout 25
Chapter 5: Essential Equipment for Beginners 32
Chapter 6: Upgrading to Intermediate Equipment 39
Chapter 7: Advanced Equipment Options 46
Chapter 8: Finding Affordable Equipment 54
Chapter 9: DIY Gym Equipment Projects 61
Chapter 10: Safety Considerations 68
Chapter 11: Organizing Your Home Gym 75
Chapter 12: Maintenance and Cleaning 83
Chapter 13: Creating a Workout Plan 90
Chapter 14: Cardio Training at Home 98
Chapter 15: Strength Training at Home 106
Chapter 16: Flexibility and Mobility Exercises 115
Chapter 17: Tracking Your Progress 124
Chapter 18: Staying Motivated 130
Chapter 19: Overcoming Common Challenges 137
Chapter 20: Expanding and Updating Your Home Gym 144
Conclusion 149

How to make a home gym

Introduction

Thank you for picking up "How to Make a Home Gym: A Comprehensive Guide to Building, Equipping, and Using Your Home Gym on a Budget." Whether you're a fitness enthusiast looking to save money, a beginner wanting to avoid the intimidating atmosphere of commercial gyms, or someone who values the convenience of working out at home, this book is for you.

Creating a home gym might seem like a big task. With so many options for equipment, different prices, and limited space, it's easy to feel confused. But it doesn't have to be hard or expensive. With the right help and a bit of creativity, you can build a home gym that fits your needs and budget.

This book will guide you through each step. We'll start by talking about the many benefits of having a home gym. Not only will you save money on gym memberships, but you'll also save time traveling and gain the freedom to work out whenever you want. Plus, a home gym gives you a private space where you can focus on your fitness goals without distractions.

Next, we'll help you look at the space you have available. Whether you have a whole basement, a spare room, or just a small corner of your living room, we'll show you how to make the most of it. Planning your layout is important to make sure your workout area is used well, and we'll give you tips to ensure every bit of space is used efficiently.

Budgeting is another important part. Many people think that creating a home gym costs a lot of money, but that's not always true. We'll help you set a budget and find quality equipment at good prices. From basic beginner gear to more advanced equipment, we'll cover everything you need to know to make smart choices.

We'll also look at DIY projects for those who like building things. Making your own equipment can save money and be a fun way to customize your gym. Plus, it adds a personal touch to your workout space.

Safety is very important in any gym, and a home gym is no different. We'll talk about how to create a safe workout environment, including keeping your equipment in good shape and preventing injuries. A well-organized and clean gym is not only safer but also more inviting, so we'll share tips on keeping your space tidy and useful.

Once your gym is set up, it's time to focus on your workouts. We'll help you create a balanced workout plan that includes cardio, strength training, and flexibility exercises. Whether you're a beginner or an experienced athlete, we'll offer routines and tips to help you reach your fitness goals.

Staying motivated can be tough, especially when working out alone. We'll talk about common obstacles and provide ways to keep your motivation and track your progress. A home gym should grow with you, so we'll also discuss ways to expand and update your gym as your fitness journey continues.

Finally, we'll provide resources for further reading and learning. The world of fitness is always changing, and staying informed is key to long-term success.

By the end of this book, you'll have the knowledge and confidence to create a home gym that suits your needs and budget. More importantly, you'll be ready to make the most of your new workout space, helping you lead a healthier, happier life.

Chapter 1: Benefits of a Home Gym

Imagine waking up and not having to rush to the gym. No need to worry about crowded spaces, waiting for equipment, or dealing with other people's schedules. With a home gym, your workout is always on your terms. One of the biggest benefits of a home gym is the convenience. You can exercise whenever you want, whether it's early in the morning, during a lunch break, or late at night. There's no need to worry about gym hours or travel time. Just step into your workout space and get started.

Another great advantage is the privacy. Many people feel self-conscious working out in front of others, especially when trying new exercises or using unfamiliar equipment. In your own home gym, you can exercise without any judgment or pressure. This can make your workouts more enjoyable and effective because you can focus solely on your fitness goals.

Having a home gym can also save you money. Gym memberships can be expensive, especially if you factor in the costs of traveling to and from the gym. While there is an initial investment in setting up your home gym, it can be much more cost-effective in the long run. You won't have to pay monthly fees, and you can buy equipment that fits your budget. Plus, with the right choices, your equipment can last for many years.

Another benefit is the ability to personalize your workout environment. In a commercial gym, you have to deal with whatever music is playing, the temperature settings, and the overall atmosphere. But in your home gym, you have complete control. You can play your favorite music, adjust the temperature to your liking, and create a space that motivates you. Whether you want bright, energizing colors or a calm, zen-like atmosphere, you can set up your gym to be the perfect workout haven.

Working out at home can also lead to more consistent exercise habits. Since the gym is just a few steps away, it's easier to fit workouts into your daily routine. You're more likely to stick to your fitness plan when you don't have to go out of your way to get to the gym. This consistency is key to seeing results and reaching your fitness goals.

A home gym is also great for families. Everyone can use it, from kids to adults. You can set a great example for your children by showing them the importance of regular exercise. Plus, working out together can be a fun family activity. It encourages a healthy lifestyle for everyone in the household.

Safety is another important benefit. In a public gym, you might worry about germs, especially on shared equipment. In your own home gym, you control the cleanliness. You can ensure that your space is clean and hygienic, giving you peace of mind as you work out.

Furthermore, a home gym eliminates the need to wait for equipment. In busy gyms, it's common to have to wait your turn for popular machines or weights. This can interrupt your workout flow and waste time. At home, everything is available to you whenever you need it, allowing for a more efficient and uninterrupted workout.

Finally, a home gym can be a great stress reliever. Life can be hectic, and finding time to unwind is crucial. Having a dedicated space to exercise at home makes it easier to incorporate stress-relief techniques like yoga or meditation into your routine. Exercise is a proven way to reduce stress, and having a home gym ensures that you always have a place to go when you need to clear your mind and focus on your well-being.

There are numerous benefits to having a home gym. It offers convenience, privacy, cost savings, and a personalized workout environment. It helps you stay consistent with your fitness routine and sets a positive example for your family. It also provides a safe, clean, and stress-free space to focus on your health. With all these advantages, it's easy to see why creating a home gym is a smart and rewarding investment in your fitness journey.

Chapter 2: Assessing Your Space

Before you start buying equipment and setting up your home gym, it's important to take a good look at the space you have available. The first step in building your home gym is assessing your space to ensure you can create a functional and enjoyable workout area.

Begin by choosing the best spot for your gym. Think about the different areas in your home. Do you have a spare room, a basement, a garage, or even a large closet that can be transformed into a workout space? If you don't have a dedicated room, don't worry. You can still create a great gym in a corner of your living room, bedroom, or even on a covered patio. The key is to find a spot where you feel comfortable and motivated to work out.

Once you've chosen a spot, measure the space. Knowing the exact dimensions will help you plan your gym layout and decide what equipment will fit. Measure the length, width, and height of the area. Make sure to note any obstacles like windows, doors, and low ceilings. This information will be crucial when you're selecting equipment and arranging your space.

Next, consider the flooring. The type of flooring in your workout area is important for both safety and comfort. If you're using a basement or garage, you might have concrete floors, which can be hard on your joints. Investing in some gym mats or rubber flooring can make a big difference. These mats not only protect your floors but also provide a cushioned surface for exercises like jumping or weightlifting. If you're setting up your gym in a room with carpet, hardwood, or tile floors, you can still use gym mats to create a more suitable workout surface.

Think about the lighting in your chosen space. Good lighting is essential for a home gym. Natural light is best, so if you have windows, make sure they are not blocked. If natural light is limited, consider adding bright, adjustable lighting to keep your workout area well-lit.

Proper lighting helps create a positive and energetic atmosphere, making your workouts more enjoyable.

Ventilation is another important factor. Working out can make you sweat, so it's important to have good airflow. If your space has windows, open them during your workout to let in fresh air. If windows are not an option, consider using fans or a portable air conditioner to keep the area cool and comfortable. Proper ventilation not only makes your workout more pleasant but also helps keep the air fresh and reduces the buildup of odors.

Storage is something you need to plan for as well. Think about where you'll store your equipment when it's not in use. Having a clutter-free workout space is important for safety and efficiency. You can use shelves, storage bins, or hooks on the wall to keep everything organized. If you have limited space, look for equipment that can be easily folded and stored away, like collapsible benches or resistance bands that can hang on a hook.

Noise is another aspect to consider. Think about the people who live with you or your neighbors. If you're planning to do high-intensity workouts or use heavy weights, it might create noise. If possible, choose a space where the noise won't disturb others. You can also add some noise-reducing mats or carpets to help minimize the sound.

Once you've assessed your space and considered these factors, it's time to think about the layout. Picture how you want your home gym to look. Plan where you'll place each piece of equipment. Leave enough room for movement and exercises that don't require equipment, like stretching or bodyweight exercises. Creating a functional layout helps you move smoothly from one exercise to the next and makes your workouts more efficient.

Lastly, think about the atmosphere you want to create. Your home gym should be a place that motivates you and makes you feel good. Consider adding personal touches like motivational posters, mirrors, or a sound system for your favorite workout music. These elements can make your gym a more inviting and inspiring place to exercise.

Assessing your space is a crucial step in creating a home gym. By carefully considering the available area, measuring dimensions, and thinking about flooring, lighting, ventilation, storage, noise, layout, and atmosphere, you can transform any space into a functional and enjoyable workout area. Taking the time to plan and organize your gym will ensure that you have a space that meets your needs and helps you stay motivated on your fitness journey.

Chapter 3: Setting Your Budget

Creating a home gym is an exciting project, but before you start buying equipment, it's important to set a budget. Setting a budget ensures that you can create a functional gym without overspending. It helps you make smart choices and find the best value for your money.

First, think about how much you can afford to spend. Look at your finances and decide on a realistic amount that won't put a strain on your budget. Remember, you don't need to buy everything all at once. You can start with the essentials and gradually add more equipment over time.

Next, consider what equipment you need the most. Think about your fitness goals and the types of exercises you enjoy. If you're just starting out, you might not need a lot of equipment. A few basic items like dumbbells, resistance bands, and a yoga mat can be enough to get you started. As you progress, you can invest in more specialized equipment like a treadmill, a weight bench, or a set of kettlebells.

Do some research to get an idea of the costs. Look at different stores, both online and in person, to compare prices. Keep an eye out for sales, discounts, and second-hand options. Many people sell lightly used gym equipment at a fraction of the cost of new items. Websites like Craigslist, eBay, and Facebook Marketplace can be great places to find deals.

Prioritize quality over quantity. It's better to have a few high-quality pieces of equipment that will last a long time than a lot of cheap items that might break quickly. Look for well-known brands with good reviews. Quality equipment is not only more durable but also safer to use.

Consider multifunctional equipment. Some pieces of equipment can be used for a variety of exercises, saving you money and space. For example, adjustable dumbbells can replace a whole set of fixed-weight dumbbells and a bench with adjustable angles can be used for different types of exercises. These items can help you get the most out of your budget.

DIY options can also help you save money. If you enjoy building things, consider making some of your own gym equipment. Simple items like plyometric boxes, squat racks, and pull-up bars can be made with basic materials and tools. There are plenty of online tutorials and plans to help you get started. DIY projects can be a fun and cost-effective way to customize your gym.

Think about the long-term costs as well. Some equipment, like treadmills and exercise bikes, might require maintenance or replacement parts over time. Factor these potential costs into your budget. Also, consider any additional items you might need, like gym mats, storage racks, or fans. These small items can add up, so it's important to include them in your overall budget.

Don't forget about your workout attire and accessories. Comfortable workout clothes, good shoes, and items like water bottles, towels, and a timer can make your workouts more enjoyable.

While these might not be major expenses, they are worth considering when setting your budget.

It's also a good idea to set aside a small portion of your budget for unexpected expenses. Sometimes, you might find a piece of equipment that you really want or need that wasn't part of your original plan. Having a little extra money set aside can give you the flexibility to make those purchases without going over budget.

Finally, be patient and flexible. Building your home gym is a process, and it's okay if it takes time to find the perfect equipment at the right price. Keep an eye on your budget and make adjustments as needed. Sometimes, you might find a great deal or realize you don't need as much equipment as you thought.

Setting a budget is a crucial step in creating your home gym. By determining how much you can afford, prioritizing your needs, doing research, and considering DIY options, you can create a functional and enjoyable workout space without overspending. Remember to prioritize quality, think about long-term costs, and be patient as you build your gym. With careful planning and smart choices, you can create a home gym that meets your fitness goals and fits your budget.

Chapter 4: Planning Your Home Gym Layout

Now that you have assessed your space and set a budget, it's time to plan your home gym layout. A well-planned layout will make your workouts more efficient and enjoyable. It will ensure you have enough room to move around and that your equipment is organized and easily accessible.

Start by visualizing your space. Picture how you want your home gym to look. Think about the different types of exercises you plan to do and the equipment you need. This will help you decide where everything should go. Remember to keep your fitness goals in mind. If you plan to do a lot of cardio, you'll need space for a treadmill or exercise bike. If strength training is your focus, you'll need room for weights and a bench.

Begin by placing the largest pieces of equipment first. These items, like treadmills, weight benches, or power racks, will take up the most space, so it's important to position them carefully. Place them in areas where they won't block walkways or limit your movement. Consider putting large machines near walls or in corners to maximize open space in the center of the room.

Next, think about the flow of your workout. You want to move smoothly from one exercise to the next without having to rearrange equipment or navigate around obstacles. For example, if you plan to do a circuit workout, arrange your equipment in the order you'll use it. This will make your workout more efficient and help you stay focused.

Consider creating different zones in your home gym. Having designated areas for different types of workouts can help keep your space organized and make it easier to transition between exercises. For example, you might have a cardio zone with your treadmill and exercise bike, a strength training zone with weights and a bench, and a stretching or yoga zone with mats and resistance bands. This can also help create a more professional and motivating workout environment.

Make sure to leave enough open space for bodyweight exercises and stretching. These activities don't require any equipment, but they do need enough room to move freely. A clear, open area in the center of your gym is ideal for exercises like lunges, push-ups, and yoga. This space can also be used for warm-ups and cool-downs.

Think about the height of your equipment as well. Some machines and exercises might require more vertical space. For example, if you have a pull-up bar or plan to do overhead lifts, make sure your ceiling is high enough to accommodate these activities. If your space has low ceilings, you might need to adjust your plans or choose different exercises.

Lighting is another important factor in your gym layout. Good lighting can make your space more inviting and help you stay focused during your workouts. If possible, position your equipment near windows to take advantage of natural light. If natural light is limited, make sure you have enough artificial lighting to keep the space bright. Consider using adjustable or dimmable lights so you can create the right atmosphere for different types of workouts.

Storage is key to keeping your home gym organized and clutter-free. Plan where you'll store your equipment when it's not in use. Shelves, storage bins, and hooks can help keep everything tidy and easily accessible. For example, you can use a rack to store your dumbbells, a bin for resistance bands, and hooks on the wall for jump ropes and yoga mats. If you have limited space, look for equipment that can be folded or stored away easily.

Mirrors can be a valuable addition to your home gym. They allow you to check your form and technique while exercising, helping you avoid injuries and improve your performance. Mirrors also make the space feel larger and brighter. Consider placing a large mirror on one wall, or use smaller mirrors strategically around the room.

Personal touches can make your gym a more enjoyable place to work out. Think about what motivates you and makes you feel good. This could be anything from motivational posters and artwork to plants and a sound system for your favorite workout music. These elements can help create a positive and inspiring atmosphere that keeps you motivated.

Safety should always be a priority in your home gym. Make sure there is enough space around each piece of equipment to move safely. Avoid placing equipment too close to walls or other obstacles that could cause accidents. Keep the floor clear of clutter and ensure that your equipment is in good condition and properly maintained.

Finally, don't be afraid to make adjustments as you go. As you start using your home gym, you might find that some things don't work as well as you thought. Be flexible and willing to rearrange your layout to better suit your needs. Your home gym should be a dynamic space that evolves with your fitness journey.

Planning your home gym layout is an important step in creating a functional and enjoyable workout space. By visualizing your space, placing large equipment first, creating workout zones, leaving open space, considering lighting and storage, adding personal touches, and prioritizing safety, you can design a gym that meets your needs and keeps you motivated. With a well-planned layout, your home gym will be a place where you look forward to working out and reaching your fitness goals.

Chapter 5: Essential Equipment for Beginners

When starting your home gym, it's important to choose the right equipment. As a beginner, you don't need to buy everything at once. Focus on getting a few key items that will help you start your fitness journey. These essential pieces of equipment will allow you to perform a wide range of exercises, helping you build strength, improve your cardio, and increase your flexibility.

One of the most versatile and essential pieces of equipment for any home gym is a set of dumbbells. Dumbbells are great for strength training and can be used for a variety of exercises, from bicep curls to shoulder presses to lunges. If you're just starting out, you might want to get a set of adjustable dumbbells. These allow you to change the weight easily, so you don't need multiple sets taking up space. Start with a weight that feels challenging but manageable, and increase it as you get stronger.

A yoga mat is another must-have item. It's not just for yoga; a good mat provides a comfortable surface for stretching, bodyweight exercises, and floor-based workouts like Pilates. It also helps protect your joints from hard floors and prevents slipping. Look for a mat that is thick enough to provide cushioning but not so thick that it's difficult to balance on.

Resistance bands are a great addition to your beginner's equipment list. They are inexpensive, lightweight, and can be used for a variety of exercises to target different muscle groups. Resistance bands are especially good for strength training and flexibility exercises. They come in different resistance levels, so you can start with a lighter band and progress to heavier ones as you get stronger.

A stability ball, also known as an exercise ball, is a useful tool for core workouts and balance training. You can use it for exercises like crunches, and planks, and even as a bench for dumbbell exercises. The instability of the ball forces your core muscles to work harder, which helps improve your balance and stability. Make sure to choose a ball that is the right size for your height.

A jump rope is a simple but effective piece of equipment for cardio workouts. It's great for getting your heart rate up and burning calories. Jumping rope can also improve your coordination and agility. It's a low-cost, high-impact workout that you can do almost anywhere. Plus, it's easy to store, making it perfect for a home gym.

A set of resistance tubes with handles can be a great alternative to traditional weights. These tubes are portable and can be used to perform a variety of exercises that target different muscle groups. They are especially useful for upper-body workouts, like chest presses, rows, and shoulder raises. Resistance tubes come in different tension levels, so you can choose the right level for your fitness level and goals.

A kettlebell is another versatile piece of equipment that is great for beginners. Kettlebells can be used for a range of exercises, from swings to squats to presses. They are particularly good for functional training, which involves movements that mimic everyday activities. Start with a lighter weight and gradually increase as you become more comfortable with the exercises.

An exercise bench is a useful addition to your home gym, especially if you plan to do a lot of strength training. A bench can be used for a variety of exercises, including bench presses, step-ups, and tricep dips. If space is an issue, look for a foldable bench that can be easily stored when not in use.

A foam roller is an essential tool for recovery and muscle maintenance. Foam rolling helps release muscle tightness, improve flexibility, and reduce soreness. It's like giving yourself a massage, which can help you recover faster from your workouts. Foam rollers come in different densities, so choose one that provides the right amount of pressure for your needs.

A set of ankle weights can add an extra challenge to your lower body workouts. They are great for exercises like leg lifts, glute bridges, and even walking. Ankle weights help increase the intensity of your workouts and build strength in your legs and glutes. Start with lighter weights and gradually increase as you get stronger.

Lastly, consider adding a fitness tracker or a simple timer to your home gym. Tracking your workouts can help you stay motivated and monitor your progress. A fitness tracker can provide valuable insights into your activity levels, heart rate, and calories burned. If a fitness tracker is out of your budget, a basic timer or stopwatch can help you keep track of your workout intervals and rest periods.

Starting your home gym with essential equipment doesn't have to be overwhelming or expensive. By focusing on a few key items like dumbbells, a yoga mat, resistance bands, a stability ball, a jump rope, resistance tubes, a kettlebell, an exercise bench, a foam roller, ankle weights, and a fitness tracker or timer, you can create a versatile and effective workout space. These pieces of equipment will help you build strength, improve your cardio, and increase your flexibility, setting a solid foundation for your fitness journey. As you progress, you can always add more equipment to suit your evolving fitness needs.

Chapter 6: Upgrading to Intermediate Equipment

Once you've been working out regularly and feel comfortable with your beginner equipment, it might be time to consider upgrading to intermediate equipment. This next level of gear can help you challenge yourself more, diversify your workouts, and continue making progress toward your fitness goals.

A good place to start is with a barbell and weight plates. Barbells allow you to lift heavier weights and perform a wider range of exercises like squats, deadlifts, and bench presses. These compound movements work for multiple muscle groups at once, making your workouts more efficient and effective. When choosing a barbell, look for one that fits your strength level and workout space. Olympic barbells are a standard choice, but if you have limited space, a shorter barbell might be more practical. You'll also need weight plates that can be added or removed to adjust the weight as needed.

Another useful piece of intermediate equipment is a squat rack or power rack. This rack provides safety and support when lifting heavy weights, especially for exercises like squats and bench presses. It usually comes with adjustable hooks and safety bars, allowing you to customize it to your height and workout needs. A squat rack can also be used for pull-ups and other bodyweight exercises, making it a versatile addition to your home gym.

If you enjoy cardio workouts, consider upgrading to a treadmill or an exercise bike. While jump ropes are great for cardio, a treadmill or bike can offer more variety and challenge. Treadmills allow you to walk, jog, or run at different speeds and inclines, simulating outdoor terrain. Exercise bikes provide a low-impact workout that's easy on the joints, with options for different resistance levels to match your fitness level. Both machines are great for improving cardiovascular health and burning calories.

A rowing machine is another excellent piece of intermediate cardio equipment. Rowing provides a full-body workout, engaging your legs, core, and upper body all at once. It's also a low-impact exercise, making it suitable for people with joint issues. Rowing machines come with adjustable resistance levels, allowing you to increase the intensity as you get stronger.

For strength training, consider adding a cable machine to your gym. Cable machines use pulleys and adjustable weights to provide constant resistance throughout your movements. They are great for targeting specific muscle groups and adding variety to your workouts. Exercises like cable rows, chest flyes, and tricep pushdowns can all be performed on a cable machine. They also allow for a greater range of motion and can help improve your stability and coordination.

If you have the space, a multi-gym machine can be a valuable investment. Multi-gym machines combine several different exercise stations into one piece of equipment. This can include a chest press, leg press, lat pulldown, and more. A multi-gym provides a comprehensive workout and is ideal for people who want to perform a variety of exercises without needing multiple machines.

Kettlebells are another great addition to your intermediate equipment. While you might already have one or two from your beginner setup, consider getting a set with different weights. Kettlebells are excellent for dynamic movements like swings, cleans, and snatches. These exercises build strength, endurance, and power. Kettlebells also help improve your grip strength and coordination.

Upgrading your resistance bands to heavier-duty versions can also provide more challenge. Look for bands with higher resistance levels or consider adding loop bands, which are great for lower body exercises like squats and leg lifts. These bands are versatile, portable, and can add a new dimension to your strength training routine.

A medicine ball can be a fun and effective addition to your home gym. Medicine balls come in various weights and can be used for exercises like slams, throws, and twists. They are great for building explosive power, core strength, and improving your overall athleticism. Medicine balls also add variety to your workouts, keeping them interesting and challenging.

If flexibility and recovery are important to you, consider upgrading to a massage gun. Massage guns provide deep-tissue massage, helping to relieve muscle soreness and improve recovery times. They are especially useful after intense workouts or for targeting tight, knotted muscles. A massage gun can help keep your muscles healthy and ready for your next workout.

Lastly, think about improving your gym environment with some additional accessories. A larger mirror can help you check your form and make adjustments as needed. Better lighting can enhance the atmosphere and make your space more inviting. You might also want to invest in a sound system or a set of Bluetooth speakers to play your favorite workout music. These upgrades can create a more motivating and enjoyable workout environment.

Upgrading to intermediate equipment can take your home gym and workouts to the next level. By adding items like a barbell and weight plates, squat rack, treadmill, rowing machine, cable machine, multi-gym, kettlebells, heavier resistance bands, medicine ball, massage gun, and improving your gym environment, you can continue to challenge yourself and make progress toward your fitness goals. These upgrades will provide more variety, increase the intensity of your workouts, and keep you motivated on your fitness journey.

Chapter 7: Advanced Equipment Options

As you continue to progress in your fitness journey, you might find yourself ready to take your home gym to the next level with advanced equipment. These items can provide more specialized workouts, target specific muscle groups, and help you achieve peak performance. Whether you're aiming to build more muscle, improve your endurance, or enhance your overall athleticism, advanced equipment can offer the variety and challenge you need.

One of the most popular pieces of advanced equipment is a power rack with attachments. A power rack is a versatile piece of equipment that allows you to perform a wide range of exercises safely. You can use it for heavy lifting, such as squats, bench presses, and deadlifts, with the added security of adjustable safety bars. Many power racks also come with attachments for pull-ups, dip bars, and even landmine attachments for rotational exercises. This equipment is essential for anyone serious about strength training.

If you're looking to enhance your cardio workouts, consider adding a commercial-grade treadmill or an elliptical machine to your gym. A commercial-grade treadmill offers more features and durability compared to standard home treadmills. It often comes with advanced settings for speed, incline, and pre-programmed workouts. An elliptical machine provides a low-impact cardio workout that engages both the upper and lower body. It's excellent for improving cardiovascular health and burning calories without putting too much strain on your joints.

A rowing machine, particularly a water rower or an air rower, is another fantastic addition for advanced cardio training. These machines simulate the action of rowing on water, providing a full-body workout that is both challenging and low-impact. Water rowers use water resistance, creating a smooth and natural rowing motion. Air rowers use a fan to create resistance, which increases with your rowing intensity. Both options are great for building endurance, strength, and improving your cardiovascular fitness.

For those focused on strength and muscle building, a set of Olympic weightlifting bars and bumper plates is a valuable investment. Olympic bars are designed to handle heavier weights and more intense lifting routines. Bumper plates are made of dense rubber, allowing them to be dropped safely during exercises like snatches and clean and jerks. This setup is ideal for anyone looking to perform Olympic lifts and other high-intensity strength training exercises.

A cable crossover machine is another excellent piece of advanced equipment. This machine features two adjustable pulleys that allow you to perform a wide variety of exercises targeting different muscle groups. It's perfect for isolation exercises and functional training, helping you improve your strength, stability, and coordination. With a cable crossover machine, you can perform exercises like cable flyes, tricep pushdowns, and cable rows with ease.

For advanced bodyweight training, consider adding a set of gymnastic rings or a TRX suspension trainer to your home gym. Gymnastic rings allow you to perform a variety of challenging exercises that build strength, stability, and coordination. Exercises like ring dips, muscle-ups, and front levers require significant upper body and core strength. A TRX suspension trainer uses your body weight for resistance, providing a full-body workout that can be adjusted for different difficulty levels. Both options are excellent for functional training and building a strong, balanced body.

A plyometric box is a great addition for those interested in explosive power and agility training. Plyometric boxes are used for exercises like box jumps, step-ups, and depth jumps. These exercises help improve your explosive strength, speed, and overall athleticism. Plyometric training is beneficial for athletes in various sports and anyone looking to enhance their performance.

A leg press machine is another valuable piece of equipment for those focused on lower body strength. The leg press allows you to target your quadriceps, hamstrings, and glutes with heavy weights in a controlled manner. It's a great alternative to squats, especially for those who might have difficulty with free-weight exercises due to balance or flexibility issues.

For recovery and mobility, consider investing in an advanced foam roller or a massage chair. An advanced foam roller, such as a vibrating roller, can provide deeper muscle relief and improve circulation. These rollers come with different intensity levels to suit your needs. A massage chair offers a luxurious way to relax and recover after intense workouts. It can help reduce muscle tension, improve blood flow, and accelerate recovery.

If you're into functional and cross-training, a battle rope can be an exciting addition. Battle ropes are used for high-intensity interval training (HIIT) and help build strength, endurance, and power. They are great for upper-body workouts and cardiovascular conditioning. Exercises like rope slams, waves, and pulls are effective and fun ways to challenge yourself.

Lastly, consider adding a smart fitness mirror to your home gym. These mirrors have built-in screens that provide virtual training sessions, real-time feedback, and a wide range of workouts. They can connect to fitness apps and track your progress, making it easier to stay motivated and achieve your fitness goals. A smart fitness mirror combines technology and fitness, offering a modern and interactive workout experience.

Upgrading to advanced equipment can significantly enhance your home gym and take your workouts to new heights. By adding items like a power rack with attachments, commercial-grade treadmill, rowing machine, Olympic weightlifting bars and bumper plates, cable crossover machine, gymnastic rings or TRX suspension trainer, plyometric box, leg press machine, advanced foam roller or massage chair, battle rope, and a smart fitness mirror, you can create a comprehensive and dynamic workout space. These advanced pieces of equipment will provide the variety, challenge, and motivation needed to continue progressing in your fitness journey and achieving your goals.

Chapter 8: Finding Affordable Equipment

Creating a home gym can be a big investment, but it doesn't have to break the bank. With a bit of creativity and smart shopping, you can find affordable equipment that suits your needs and budget. Finding the right deals and making cost-effective choices will allow you to build a functional and enjoyable workout space without spending too much money.

One of the best ways to find affordable equipment is to look for used items. Many people sell their gently used gym equipment at a fraction of the cost of new items. You can find great deals on websites like Craigslist, Facebook Marketplace, eBay, and local classified ads. Check these sites regularly for new listings, and be ready to act quickly when you find a good deal. Visiting garage sales and thrift stores can also lead to unexpected finds. Always inspect the equipment carefully to ensure it's in good condition before making a purchase.

Another option is to buy refurbished equipment. Many fitness stores and online retailers offer refurbished machines like treadmills, exercise bikes, and ellipticals at a significant discount. These items have been repaired and tested to ensure they work like new. Buying refurbished can be a great way to get high-quality equipment at a lower price. Make sure to buy from reputable sellers who offer warranties or return policies in case something goes wrong.

Discount stores and clearance sales are also excellent places to find affordable equipment. Stores like Walmart, Target, and sporting goods stores often have sales on fitness equipment, especially during certain times of the year like after New Year's or during summer sales events. Look for clearance items or end-of-season sales where you can find significant discounts on a variety of equipment. Signing up for store newsletters or following them on social media can keep you informed about upcoming sales and promotions.

Online retailers like Amazon often have competitive prices and frequent sales on fitness equipment. You can use price comparison tools or browser extensions to track price drops and find the best deals. Reading customer reviews can also help you identify which products offer the best value for money. Sometimes, lesser-known brands can offer high-quality equipment at a lower price than big-name brands.

Consider looking for package deals or bundles. Some retailers offer discounts when you buy multiple items together, such as a set of dumbbells with a weight bench or a package of resistance bands with a stability ball. These bundles can provide everything you need to get started while saving you money compared to buying each item separately.

DIY equipment is another cost-effective option. With some basic tools and materials, you can make your own gym equipment. For example, you can build a plyometric box using plywood, or create a set of parallettes with PVC pipes. There are many online tutorials and guides that can help you build various types of equipment.

Not only can DIY projects save you money, but they also allow you to customize the equipment to your specific needs and space.

Joining local community groups or fitness forums can connect you with people who are looking to sell or give away their equipment. Sometimes, people move or upgrade their gyms and are happy to pass on their old equipment for free or at a low cost. Community centers, gyms, or fitness studios might also sell used equipment when they upgrade their facilities. Keep an eye on local bulletin boards or online community boards for announcements.

Opting for multipurpose equipment can save you both money and space. Items like adjustable dumbbells, which can replace an entire rack of fixed-weight dumbbells, or a bench with adjustable angles that can be used for various exercises, are excellent choices. Look for equipment that can serve multiple functions and support a wide range of exercises.

When shopping for affordable equipment, consider what you truly need versus what would be nice to have. Start with the basics and gradually add more specialized items as your budget allows. Prioritizing essential equipment like dumbbells, resistance bands, and a yoga mat can help you get started without spending too much. As you progress in your fitness journey, you can identify additional equipment that will be most beneficial for your workouts.

Utilize free resources to complement your equipment. There are many free workout apps, YouTube channels, and online fitness communities that offer a variety of workout routines and guidance. These resources can help you make the most of the equipment you have and provide new ideas for your workouts. They can also help you learn proper form and technique, reducing the risk of injury.

Lastly, be patient and persistent. Building a home gym on a budget takes time, but with careful planning and smart shopping, you can find affordable equipment that meets your needs. Keep an eye out for deals, be open to buying used or refurbished items, and consider DIY options. Over time, you'll be able to create a fully equipped home gym that supports your fitness goals without overspending.

Finding affordable equipment for your home gym is achievable with some creativity and resourcefulness. By exploring used and refurbished options, shopping during sales, considering DIY projects, and prioritizing multipurpose equipment, you can build a functional and effective workout space on a budget. Take advantage of free resources and be patient in your search for the best deals. With the right approach, you can create a home gym that helps you stay fit and healthy without breaking the bank.

Chapter 9: DIY Gym Equipment Projects

Creating your own gym equipment can be a fun and cost-effective way to build your home gym. With some basic materials, tools, and a bit of creativity, you can make sturdy and functional equipment that meets your workout needs. DIY projects not only save money but also allow you to customize equipment to fit your space and preferences. Here are some ideas for DIY gym equipment that you can easily make at home.

One of the simplest and most useful DIY projects is a set of parallettes. Parallettes are small bars used for bodyweight exercises like dips, push-ups, and L-sits. To make them, you need PVC pipes, elbow joints, T-joints, and some PVC cement. Cut the PVC pipes to the desired length for the base and the handles. Assemble the pieces using the T-joints for the base and elbow joints for the handles. Glue everything together with PVC cement for extra stability. Parallettes are lightweight, portable, and great for strengthening your upper body and core.

Another straightforward project is a sandbag. Sandbags are versatile and can be used for lifting, carrying, throwing, and more. To make a sandbag, you need a sturdy duffel bag or an old gym bag, heavy-duty garbage bags, and duct tape. Fill the garbage bags with sand or gravel, seal them tightly with duct tape, and place them inside the duffel bag. Make sure the sandbags are well-sealed to prevent leaks. You can adjust the weight by adding or removing sandbags. Sandbags are excellent for functional training, building strength, and improving endurance.

A homemade medicine ball is another useful piece of equipment. For this project, you need an old basketball, a funnel, sand or rice, and duct tape. Cut a small slit in the basketball, insert the funnel, and fill the ball with sand or rice until it reaches the desired weight. Seal the slit with strong adhesive or duct tape. You can use the medicine ball for various exercises like slams, throws, and twists, which help build explosive power, core strength, and overall fitness.

If you need a sturdy box for plyometric exercises, you can build a plyometric box using plywood and screws. Cut the plywood into six pieces: two pieces for the top and bottom, and four pieces for the sides. Assemble the box by screwing the sides to the bottom piece, then attach the top piece. Make sure the edges are smooth to avoid splinters. A plyometric box is perfect for exercises like box jumps, step-ups, and depth jumps, which enhance your explosive power and agility.

A DIY pull-up bar can be made with galvanized steel pipes and fittings. You need two long pipes for the uprights, one shorter pipe for the bar, four-floor flanges, and eight screws. Attach the floor flanges to the ends of the uprights and the bar. Secure the flanges to a sturdy wall or ceiling with screws, making sure the bar is at a comfortable height for you. Pull-ups are great for building upper body and back strength and having a pull-up bar at home makes it easy to practice regularly.

For a simple yet effective piece of equipment, consider making a battle rope. You need a long piece of thick rope, about 40-50 feet, and some duct tape. Wrap the ends of the rope with duct tape to prevent fraying. You can use the battle rope for high-intensity interval training (HIIT) exercises like rope slams, waves, and pulls. Battle ropes provide a full-body workout, improving strength, endurance, and cardiovascular fitness.

If you want to add resistance to your workouts, you can make your own resistance bands using bicycle inner tubes. Cut the inner tubes to the desired length, and secure the ends with strong knots or zip ties. You can also attach handles made from PVC pipes for a more comfortable grip. These DIY resistance bands are great for strength training, stretching, and mobility exercises.

A homemade weighted vest can enhance your bodyweight exercises and add intensity to your workouts. To make a weighted vest, you need a sturdy vest with multiple pockets and some small weights like sandbags or metal plates. Fill the pockets with the weights, distributing them evenly for balance. A weighted vest is useful for exercises like push-ups, pull-ups, and running, helping to build strength and endurance.

Building a stability ball stand is another practical DIY project. Stability balls are excellent for core workouts, but they can roll around when not in use. To make a stand, you need a wooden board and four wooden dowels. Cut the dowels to the same height and attach them to the corners of the board to create a square frame. Place the stability ball inside the frame to keep it from rolling away. This simple stand keeps your gym organized and makes your stability ball easily accessible.

If you need a sturdy bench for weightlifting, you can build a weight bench using plywood, wooden beams, and screws. Cut the plywood to the desired size for the bench top and attach it to a frame made from wooden beams. Reinforce the frame with additional beams for extra stability. Cover the bench top with a layer of foam for padding and secure it with a durable fabric. A homemade weight bench is great for exercises like bench presses, step-ups, and seated exercises.

Making your own gym equipment can be a rewarding and economical way to build your home gym. Projects like parallettes, sandbags, medicine balls, plyometric boxes, pull-up bars, battle ropes, resistance bands, weighted vests, stability ball stands, and weight benches can be made with simple materials and tools. These DIY projects not only save money but also allow you to customize your equipment to fit your needs and space. With a bit of effort and creativity, you can create a functional and effective workout environment at home.

Chapter 10: Safety Considerations

When setting up a home gym, safety should be your top priority. Making sure that your workout space is safe helps prevent injuries and ensures that you can exercise confidently. Here are some important safety considerations to keep in mind as you build and use your home gym.

First, choose a suitable location for your home gym. Look for a space that is well-ventilated and has enough room for you to move around freely. Basements, garages, and spare rooms are often good options. Make sure the floor is stable and can support the weight of your equipment. If you're setting up in a room with carpet, consider placing rubber mats or interlocking foam tiles to provide a solid and non-slip surface.

Lighting is another crucial factor. A well-lit gym helps you see what you're doing and prevents accidents. Natural light is best, but if that's not possible, install bright and even lighting. Avoid using dim or flickering lights, as they can create shadows and make it harder to see your equipment and surroundings clearly.

Organize your equipment properly to avoid clutter and tripping hazards. Keep weights, dumbbells, and other small items stored on racks or shelves when not in use. This not only keeps your gym tidy but also prevents accidents caused by stepping on or tripping over loose equipment. Make sure larger items, like treadmills or weight benches, are placed in a way that allows enough space for you to move around them safely.

Inspect your equipment regularly to ensure it is in good working condition. Check for any signs of wear and tear, such as frayed cables, loose bolts, or cracks in the frames. If you notice any damage, repair or replace the equipment before using it again. Regular maintenance extends the life of your equipment and keeps it safe to use.

Proper form and technique are essential for preventing injuries. When performing exercises, always focus on using the correct form. If you're unsure about how to do a particular exercise, look for instructional videos or consult a fitness professional. Using improper form can lead to strains, sprains, and more serious injuries over time. Start with lighter weights or lower intensity to master the movements before progressing to heavier loads.

Warming up before your workouts is another key safety practice. A proper warm-up prepares your body for exercise by increasing your heart rate and loosening your muscles. Spend at least 5-10 minutes doing light cardio, like jogging in place or jumping jacks, followed by dynamic stretches that target the muscles you'll be working. This reduces the risk of injury and helps improve your performance during the workout.

Cooling down after your workouts is equally important. Cooling down helps your body transition back to a resting state and prevents dizziness or fainting. Spend a few minutes doing light cardio, like walking, followed by static stretches to relax your muscles and improve flexibility. This also aids in recovery and reduces muscle soreness.

Hydration is crucial during exercise. Keep a water bottle nearby and take regular sips throughout your workout. Dehydration can lead to fatigue, dizziness, and even heatstroke, especially during intense exercise or in hot environments. Drinking enough water helps you stay energized and perform at your best.

Listening to your body is another vital aspect of exercising safely. Pay attention to any signs of discomfort or pain during your workouts. If you experience sharp pain, stop immediately and assess the situation. Continuing to exercise through pain can lead to more severe injuries. It's important to know the difference between the normal discomfort of exertion and the pain of an injury.

Using proper footwear is also important for your safety. Wear shoes that provide adequate support and cushioning for your activities. Running shoes are great for cardio exercises, while cross-training shoes offer better stability for weightlifting and other dynamic movements. Avoid exercising in worn-out or inappropriate footwear, as this can lead to injuries.

If you're lifting heavy weights, consider having a spotter or using safety equipment like a power rack with safety bars. A spotter can assist you if you struggle with a lift, while safety bars can catch the weight if you need to drop it. This is especially important for exercises like squats and bench presses, where losing control of the weight can be dangerous.

In case of an emergency, have a plan in place. Keep a first aid kit in your home gym, and know how to use it. Include items like bandages, antiseptic wipes, ice packs, and pain relievers. It's also a good idea to have a phone nearby in case you need to call for help.

Lastly, consider getting professional advice if you're new to exercise or trying something unfamiliar. A personal trainer can provide guidance on proper form, workout routines, and equipment use. They can also help you develop a plan that suits your fitness level and goals, ensuring you exercise safely and effectively.

Ensuring safety in your home gym is essential for preventing injuries and making your workouts enjoyable. By choosing a suitable location, organizing your equipment, maintaining proper form, warming up and cooling down, staying hydrated, listening to your body, wearing appropriate footwear, using safety measures, and having an emergency plan, you can create a safe and effective workout environment. Taking these precautions helps you stay healthy and motivated on your fitness journey.

Chapter 11: Organizing Your Home Gym

Creating a home gym is exciting, but keeping it organized is just as important. A well-organized gym makes your workouts smoother and more enjoyable. It helps you find your equipment easily and ensures a safe and tidy workout space. Here are some tips on how to organize your home gym effectively.

First, think about how you want to use your space. Consider the types of exercises you'll be doing and the equipment you need. Plan the layout of your gym so that everything has a designated place. This will help you maximize your space and keep it functional. If you have a small area, focus on the essentials and look for multipurpose equipment that can be used for various exercises.

Start by organizing your larger equipment. Place items like treadmills, stationary bikes, and weight benches against the walls to keep the center of the room open. This not only saves space but also makes your gym look less cluttered. Ensure that there's enough space around each piece of equipment for you to move comfortably and safely.

For your weights and dumbbells, invest in a good storage rack. A weight rack keeps your dumbbells off the floor and organized by size, making it easy to find the weight you need. If you have limited space, consider a compact, vertical rack that holds multiple weights in a small footprint. Keep your weight plates on a plate tree or stack them neatly in a corner. This prevents them from rolling around and getting in the way.

Resistance bands and jump ropes can be hung on hooks or pegs on the wall. This keeps them untangled and easy to access. You can also use a pegboard to organize smaller equipment like resistance bands, jump ropes, and other accessories. Pegboards are customizable and allow you to arrange your equipment in a way that suits your needs.

Shelves and storage bins are great for keeping smaller items like yoga blocks, foam rollers, and fitness balls organized. Use clear bins so you can see what's inside without having to dig through them. Label the bins if needed to make finding things even easier. Place these bins on shelves to keep them off the floor and within reach.

For your yoga mat, consider getting a wall-mounted mat holder or a mat rack. This keeps your mat rolled up and out of the way when you're not using it. It also prevents it from getting dirty or damaged on the floor. If you have multiple mats or other flat items like exercise posters, a vertical storage solution can keep them neatly organized.

Keep your workout area clean and inviting by storing cleaning supplies nearby. A small caddy with disinfectant wipes, towels, and a spray bottle can help you quickly wipe down your equipment after each use. Regular cleaning not only keeps your gym looking good but also ensures that your equipment stays in good condition and free of sweat and grime.

Mirrors are a useful addition to any home gym. They help you check your form during exercises and make the space feel larger and brighter. Place mirrors on the walls where you can easily see yourself while working out. This can help you stay motivated and ensure that you're performing exercises correctly.

If you have a TV or a screen for workout videos, mount it on the wall to save space. Position it at eye level when you're standing or sitting on your equipment. This setup makes it easy to follow along with workout routines and keeps your floor space clear. You can also connect your screen to speakers for better sound quality during your workouts.

Music can be a great motivator, so consider setting up a small sound system or Bluetooth speakers in your gym. Place the speakers in spots where the sound can reach all corners of the room. This way, you can enjoy your favorite workout tunes without dealing with tangled wires or moving equipment around.

To keep track of your workouts and progress, create a dedicated space for a workout journal or a whiteboard. You can write down your goals, track your sets and reps, or plan your workout schedule. Having a visual reminder of your progress can be very motivating and help you stay on track with your fitness goals.

For those who enjoy a touch of nature, adding some plants to your home gym can make the space more pleasant and refreshing. Choose low-maintenance plants that can thrive indoors, like succulents or snake plants. Plants can improve air quality and add a bit of greenery to your workout environment.

Lighting plays a crucial role in creating an inviting workout space. If possible, maximize natural light by setting up your gym near windows. For artificial lighting, use bright, white lights that mimic daylight. Avoid dim or yellow lighting, as it can make the space feel small and dull.

Safety is key in any gym, so make sure to keep your floor clear of obstacles. Store away any items that you're not using and ensure that cables and wires are neatly managed. Tripping over loose equipment or wires can lead to injuries, so always check your space before starting your workout.

Finally, personalize your gym with motivational posters, quotes, or photos that inspire you. Creating a space that reflects your personality and fitness goals can make your gym a place you look forward to spending time in. Whether it's a favorite quote, a picture of a fitness icon, or a poster of your dream destination, personal touches can boost your motivation and make your gym feel like your own.

Organizing your home gym is essential for creating a functional and enjoyable workout space. By planning your layout, using storage solutions, keeping your area clean, and adding personal touches, you can make your gym inviting and efficient. A well-organized gym helps you focus on your workouts, stay motivated, and reach your fitness goals more effectively.

Chapter 12: Maintenance and Cleaning

Keeping your home gym clean and well-maintained is important for several reasons. It helps your equipment last longer, keeps your workout space safe, and makes your gym a more pleasant place to be. Regular maintenance and cleaning can seem like a chore, but it's worth the effort. Here's how you can keep your home gym in top shape.

First, let's talk about cleaning. After each workout, take a few minutes to wipe down your equipment. Sweat can cause rust and wear on metal parts, and it can also make your gym smell unpleasant. Use disinfectant wipes or a spray bottle with a mixture of water and mild soap. Wipe down handles, seats, benches, and any other surfaces you touched during your workout. Don't forget to clean your yoga mat and any other floor mats you use. Keeping things clean helps prevent the spread of germs and keeps your gym smelling fresh.

At least once a week, do a more thorough cleaning. Vacuum or sweep the floor to remove dust and dirt. If you have rubber mats or foam tiles, you can mop them with a mild detergent and water. Make sure the floor is completely dry before you start your next workout to avoid slipping. Dust off any shelves, racks, and equipment that you didn't use during your daily workouts. A clean gym is not only more pleasant but also healthier for you.

Now, let's move on to maintenance. Regularly checking your equipment for signs of wear and tear can prevent small problems from becoming big issues. Start by inspecting your weights and dumbbells. Look for cracks or chips, and make sure the handles are secure. If you have adjustable dumbbells, check the locking mechanisms to ensure they are working properly.

For cardio equipment like treadmills and exercise bikes, it's important to follow the manufacturer's maintenance recommendations. This usually includes lubricating moving parts, checking belts and pedals for wear, and tightening any loose bolts. For treadmills, keep the belt clean and centered. If the belt starts to slip or make noise, it might be time to adjust or replace it. Regular maintenance keeps your equipment running smoothly and extends its life.

Your weight bench and any other large pieces of equipment also need regular attention. Check the bolts and screws to make sure everything is tight. If you notice any wobbling or instability, stop using the equipment until you fix it. Look for cracks or tears in the padding, and repair or replace it if necessary. Keeping your equipment stable and in good condition helps prevent accidents and injuries.

If you use resistance bands, take a close look at them every so often. Look for any signs of fraying or cracking, especially near the handles or attachment points. Resistance bands can snap if they are worn out, which can cause injuries. Replace any bands that show signs of wear to stay safe.

Electronic equipment like heart rate monitors, fitness trackers, and any connected devices should also be checked regularly. Replace batteries as needed and keep the screens clean. Make sure any charging cables are in good condition and stored neatly to prevent damage.

To keep your gym organized and clutter-free, make it a habit to put things away after each workout. Store weights on racks, hang resistance bands on hooks and place small items like yoga blocks and foam rollers in bins or on shelves. This not only keeps your gym looking tidy but also makes it easier to find what you need for your next workout.

Consider setting a monthly schedule for more in-depth maintenance tasks. This might include checking all the bolts and screws on your equipment, lubricating moving parts, and giving your gym a deep clean. Mark these tasks on your calendar so you don't forget them. Regular maintenance and cleaning can save you money in the long run by preventing costly repairs or replacements.

Keeping your home gym well-ventilated is also important. Good airflow helps prevent mold and mildew, especially in areas where you sweat a lot. If your gym is in a basement or a room without windows, consider using a fan or a dehumidifier to improve air circulation. Opening windows when the weather is nice can also help keep the air fresh.

Another tip is to take care of your workout clothes and towels. Wash them regularly and store them in a clean, dry place. Dirty, damp clothes and towels can contribute to unpleasant odors and even mold growth in your gym. Keeping them clean and dry helps maintain a pleasant environment.

In case of any spills or accidents, clean them up immediately. Whether it's a water bottle that tipped over or a bit of sweat on the floor, dealing with it right away prevents stains and damage. Keep a small cleaning kit in your gym with towels, disinfectant spray, and a mop or broom for quick clean-ups.

Lastly, keep an eye on your gym's environment. If you notice any unusual smells, stains, or other issues, address them right away. Sometimes, small problems can indicate larger issues, like a leak or poor ventilation. Staying on top of these things helps you keep your gym in great condition.

Maintaining and cleaning your home gym is essential for keeping your workout space safe, pleasant, and functional. Regular cleaning prevents germs and odors, while routine maintenance keeps your equipment in good working order. By making these tasks a part of your routine, you can enjoy a clean and well-organized gym that supports your fitness goals for years to come.

Chapter 13: Creating a Workout Plan

Creating a workout plan is like designing a roadmap for your fitness journey. It helps you stay focused, motivated, and on track to reach your goals. Whether you're new to exercise or a seasoned athlete, having a structured plan can make a big difference in your progress. Here's how to create a workout plan that works for you.

Start by setting clear and achievable goals. Think about what you want to accomplish. Do you want to lose weight, build muscle, increase your endurance, or just feel healthier? Your goals will guide the rest of your plan. Be specific and realistic. For example, instead of saying, "I want to get fit," say, "I want to lose 10 pounds in three months" or "I want to run a 5k in under 30 minutes."

Once you have your goals, it's time to assess your current fitness level. This will help you understand where you're starting from and how much you can handle. You can do this by trying some basic exercises and noting how you feel. For example, see how many push-ups you can do, how long you can hold a plank, or how far you can run without stopping. Be honest with yourself about your strengths and areas that need improvement.

Now, decide how many days a week you can commit to working out. Consistency is key, so choose a schedule that fits into your life. If you're just starting out, three to four days a week is a good goal. If you're more experienced, you might aim for five to six days. Make sure to include rest days in your plan. Your body needs time to recover and get stronger.

Next, plan the types of workouts you'll do each day. A well-rounded workout plan includes a mix of cardio, strength training, and flexibility exercises. Cardio, like running, biking, or dancing, helps improve your heart health and burn calories. Strength training, such as lifting weights or doing bodyweight exercises, builds muscle and boosts your metabolism. Flexibility exercises, like stretching or yoga, help keep your muscles and joints healthy and reduce the risk of injury.

Here's a sample weekly workout plan to get you started:

- Monday: Cardio - 30 minutes of running or brisk walking
- Tuesday: Strength training - Full body workout with weights or bodyweight exercises
- Wednesday: Rest or light activity like a gentle walk or stretching
- Thursday: Cardio - 30 minutes of biking or a dance class
- Friday: Strength training - Focus on upper body exercises
- Saturday: Cardio - 30 minutes of swimming or hiking
- Sunday: Flexibility - Yoga or stretching routine

When planning your strength training workouts, divide your exercises into different muscle groups. For example, one day you might focus on your upper body (arms, chest, back), and another day on your lower body (legs, glutes). This ensures that all your major muscles get worked out without overloading any single group.

It's also important to vary your workouts to keep them interesting and challenging. Doing the same exercises every day can lead to boredom and plateaus in your progress. Mix things up by trying new activities, changing the intensity, or increasing the weights you use. Variety keeps your body guessing and helps you continue to improve.

Warm up before each workout and cool down afterward. A proper warm-up gets your blood flowing and prepares your muscles for exercise. This can be as simple as five to ten minutes of light cardio, like jogging or jumping jacks. Cooling down helps your body transition back to a resting state and can prevent stiffness and soreness. Spend a few minutes stretching the muscles you worked during your session.

Tracking your progress is another key part of a successful workout plan. Keep a workout journal or use a fitness app to record what you did each day, how you felt, and any improvements you noticed. Seeing your progress over time can be incredibly motivating and help you stay committed to your plan.

Don't forget to listen to your body. If you're feeling extremely tired, sore, or unwell, it's okay to take an extra rest day. Pushing through pain can lead to injury, which can set you back even further. It's better to take a short break and come back stronger than to risk hurting yourself.

In addition to your workouts, pay attention to your diet and hydration. Eating a balanced diet that includes plenty of fruits, vegetables, lean proteins, and whole grains gives your body the fuel it needs to perform and recover. Staying hydrated is equally important. Drink plenty of water before, during, and after your workouts to keep your energy levels up and prevent dehydration.

Getting enough sleep is also crucial. Aim for seven to nine hours of sleep each night to allow your body to recover and rebuild. Lack of sleep can affect your performance and make it harder to reach your fitness goals.

Consider getting support from others. Join a fitness class, find a workout buddy, or connect with an online fitness community. Having someone to share your journey with can make exercise more fun and provide extra motivation. You can encourage each other, share tips, and celebrate your successes together.

Finally, be patient and stay positive. Results don't happen overnight, but with consistency and effort, you will see improvements. Celebrate the small victories along the way, whether it's lifting a heavier weight, running a bit farther, or simply feeling better. Remember, the journey to fitness is a marathon, not a sprint.

Creating a workout plan involves setting clear goals, assessing your fitness level, choosing a realistic schedule, and including a variety of exercises. Warm-up and cool down properly, track your progress, listen to your body, and take care of your nutrition and sleep. Seek support and stay positive. With a well-thought-out plan, you can make steady progress and achieve your fitness goals.

Chapter 14: Cardio Training at Home

Cardio training is essential for a healthy heart, strong lungs, and overall fitness. It helps you burn calories, improve your endurance, and feel more energetic. You don't need a gym membership or fancy equipment to get a good cardio workout. You can do it all from the comfort of your home. Here's how to make cardio training at home effective and enjoyable.

Start by choosing the right space. You don't need a lot of room, just enough to move around comfortably. A living room, bedroom, or even a backyard can work. Clear the area of any furniture or obstacles that might get in your way. Make sure you have a flat, non-slip surface to exercise on. If you have a mat, lay it down to provide extra cushioning for your joints.

One of the simplest and most effective cardio exercises you can do at home is jumping jacks.

They get your heart rate up quickly and work your whole body. Start by standing with your feet together and your arms at your sides. Jump up, spreading your legs shoulder-width apart and raising your arms above your head. Jump again to return to the starting position. Repeat this for 30 seconds to a minute. As you get stronger, you can increase the time or speed.

Another great exercise is running in place. It's easy to do and doesn't require any equipment. Simply lift your knees high and pump your arms as if you're running. Try to keep a steady pace and maintain good form. Running in place is a fantastic way to boost your heart rate and build endurance. You can mix it up by doing high knees, where you lift your knees higher than usual, or butt kicks, where you kick your heels up towards your glutes.

Burpees are a more intense option that combines cardio with strength training. They work your entire body and really get your heart pumping. To do a burpee, start in a standing position. Drop into a squat, placing your hands on the floor in front of you. Jump your feet back to land in a plank position. Do a push-up, then jump your feet back to your hands. Finally, jump up with your arms raised. Repeat this sequence for 10 to 15 repetitions. Burpees are challenging, but they're incredibly effective for building strength and cardiovascular fitness.

If you prefer a lower-impact option, consider doing some marching in place. It's easier on the joints but still gets your heart rate up. Stand tall and lift one knee at a time, as if you're marching. Swing your arms to help keep your balance and increase the intensity. You can also step side to side, bringing your knees up high. Marching in place is a great way to warm up before more intense exercises or cool down afterward.

Dance is another fun way to get your cardio in. Put on your favorite music and let loose. You don't need any specific moves; just keep moving to the beat. Dancing is a great way to burn calories and improve your coordination while having fun. You can follow along with dance workout videos online or create your own routine. The key is to keep your body moving and your heart rate up.

Jump rope is a classic cardio exercise that's both fun and effective. If you have a jump rope, use it to do different jump variations. Start with basic jumps, then try alternating feet, high knees, or criss cross jumps. If you don't have a jump rope, you can mimic the movements without one. Jumping rope improves your coordination, balance, and cardiovascular health. Aim for short bursts of one to two minutes, then rest and repeat.

For a more structured workout, consider creating a circuit. A circuit involves doing several exercises in a row, with little to no rest in between. You can combine different cardio exercises to keep things interesting. For example, you might do one minute of jumping jacks, one minute of running in place, one minute of burpees, and one minute of dancing. Repeat the circuit two or three times for a full workout. Circuits keep your heart rate elevated and help you burn more calories in less time.

If you enjoy following along with workouts, there are plenty of online resources available. YouTube has countless free workout videos, ranging from beginner to advanced levels. Look for cardio workouts that match your fitness level and interests. Following a video can provide structure and motivation, especially if you're new to exercising at home.

Remember to warm up before starting your cardio workout. Spend five to ten minutes doing light activities like walking in place, gentle stretching, or easy jumping jacks. Warming up prepares your muscles and joints for more intense exercise and helps prevent injuries.

After your workout, cool down with some light stretching or slow walking. Cooling down helps your heart rate return to normal and reduces muscle soreness. Stretch the muscles you used during your workout, holding each stretch for 15 to 30 seconds. This can improve your flexibility and promote better recovery.

Staying hydrated is crucial during cardio workouts. Drink water before, during, and after your exercise session. Dehydration can make you feel tired and decrease your performance, so keep a water bottle nearby and take sips regularly.

To stay motivated, set goals for your cardio training. Maybe you want to increase the time you can do a particular exercise, or perhaps you want to try new workout videos each week. Setting goals gives you something to work towards and helps keep your workouts interesting.

Incorporating cardio into your routine doesn't mean you have to spend hours working out. Even short bursts of 10 to 15 minutes can be effective, especially if you're consistent. Find a time that works for you, whether it's in the morning, during lunch, or in the evening. Make cardio a regular part of your day, and you'll start to see and feel the benefits.

Cardio training at home is accessible, effective, and can be a lot of fun. With exercises like jumping jacks, running in place, burpees, marching, dancing, and jumping rope, you can get a great workout without any special equipment. Create circuits, follow online videos, and stay motivated with clear goals. Remember to warm up, cool down, and stay hydrated. With a little creativity and consistency, you can make cardio training a rewarding part of your fitness journey.

Chapter 15: Strength Training at Home

Strength training at home is a fantastic way to build muscle, increase your strength, and improve your overall fitness. You don't need a gym membership or expensive equipment to get started. With a few basic items and your own body weight, you can create an effective strength training routine right at home. Here's how to do it.

First, let's talk about why strength training is important. It helps you build and maintain muscle, which is essential for staying strong and healthy. It also boosts your metabolism, which helps you burn more calories even when you're not working out. Strength training improves your bone density, reducing the risk of osteoporosis. It enhances your balance and coordination, making everyday activities easier and reducing the risk of falls and injuries. Plus, it can boost your mood and energy levels.

To start, you need a few basic pieces of equipment. If you have dumbbells, resistance bands, or kettlebells, those are great. If not, you can use items you already have at home. Water bottles or canned goods can serve as makeshift weights. You can also use a sturdy chair or a step for exercises that require elevation. A yoga mat or a towel can provide some cushioning for floor exercises.

Begin with a warm-up. Spend five to ten minutes doing light cardio to get your blood flowing and your muscles ready. This can be jogging in place, jumping jacks, or even dancing. A proper warm-up helps prevent injuries and makes your workout more effective.

One of the best bodyweight exercises for strength training is the push-up. Push-ups work your chest, shoulders, triceps, and core. Start in a plank position with your hands slightly wider than shoulder-width apart. Lower your body until your chest almost touches the floor, then push back up to the starting position. Keep your body in a straight line from head to heels. If regular push-ups are too challenging, try doing them on your knees or against a wall. Aim for three sets of 10 to 15 repetitions.

Squats are another excellent bodyweight exercise. They target your legs, glutes, and core. Stand with your feet shoulder-width apart. Lower your body as if you're sitting back in a chair, keeping your chest up and your knees over your toes. Push through your heels to return to the starting position. To add resistance, hold a weight or a heavy object at your chest. Try to do three sets of 15 to 20 squats.

Lunges are great for working your legs and glutes. Stand with your feet together. Step forward with one leg and lower your body until both knees are bent at 90 degrees. Push through your front heel to return to the starting position, then repeat on the other side. For added resistance, hold weights in each hand. Do three sets of 10 to 15 lunges on each leg.

Planks are excellent for strengthening your core. Start in a push-up position but rest on your forearms instead of your hands. Keep your body in a straight line from head to heels. Hold this position for as long as you can, aiming for at least 30 seconds. As you get stronger, try to hold the plank for longer periods or add variations like lifting one leg or one arm.

For your back and biceps, try doing rows. If you have dumbbells, bend over at the waist with a slight bend in your knees. Hold a dumbbell in each hand with your arms hanging straight down. Pull the weights up towards your waist, squeezing your shoulder blades together, then lower them back down. If you don't have dumbbells, you can use water bottles or other heavy objects. Do three sets of 12 to 15 repetitions.

Tricep dips are effective for targeting the back of your arms. Sit on the edge of a chair or a step with your hands gripping the edge, fingers pointing forward. Slide your butt off the edge and lower your body until your elbows are bent at 90 degrees. Push back up to the starting position. Keep your legs bent for an easier version, or straighten them out for more of a challenge. Aim for three sets of 10 to 15 dips.

If you have resistance bands, you can use them for a variety of exercises. For example, stand on the band with your feet shoulder-width apart and hold the handles at shoulder height. Press the handles overhead to work your shoulders. For bicep curls, stand on the band and hold the handles with your palms facing up. Curl your hands up towards your shoulders, then lower them back down. Resistance bands are versatile and can add extra challenge to many exercises.

Don't forget to work on your lower back and glutes. Bridges are a great exercise for this. Lie on your back with your knees bent and your feet flat on the floor. Lift your hips towards the ceiling, squeezing your glutes at the top, then lower back down. You can make this exercise more challenging by placing a weight on your hips or doing single-leg bridges. Aim for three sets of 15 to 20 repetitions.

Include some flexibility and mobility exercises in your routine. Stretching after your workout helps your muscles recover and improves your flexibility. Focus on the major muscle groups you worked on during your strength training.

Hold each stretch for at least 15 to 30 seconds. Yoga can also be a great addition to your routine, as it combines strength, flexibility, and relaxation.

It's important to progress gradually. Start with lighter weights or fewer repetitions, and increase them as you get stronger. Listen to your body and avoid pushing through pain. Rest is crucial for muscle recovery and growth, so make sure to include rest days in your schedule. Aim for two to three days of strength training per week, with at least one day of rest in between sessions.

Stay motivated by setting goals and tracking your progress. Keep a workout journal or use an app to record your exercises, weights, and repetitions. Celebrate your achievements, no matter how small. Remember that consistency is key. It's better to do shorter, regular workouts than long, infrequent ones.

If you need guidance, there are plenty of online resources available. Follow along with workout videos, join virtual fitness classes, or use apps that provide strength training programs. Having a plan to follow can help you stay on track and ensure you're doing the exercises correctly.

Strength training at home offers flexibility and convenience. You can work out whenever it fits your schedule, and you don't have to worry about commuting to a gym. It's also a great way to set a positive example for family members and encourage them to join you.

Strength training at home is accessible and effective. With a few basic pieces of equipment and your own body weight, you can build muscle, increase strength, and improve your overall fitness. Warm up properly, focus on form, and progress gradually. Include a variety of exercises for different muscle groups, and don't forget to stretch and rest. Stay motivated by setting goals and tracking your progress. With consistency and effort, you can achieve great results right from the comfort of your home.

Chapter 16: Flexibility and Mobility Exercises

Flexibility and mobility exercises are essential for keeping your body healthy and moving well. These exercises help you stay limber, reduce the risk of injury, and improve your overall quality of life. Whether you're young or old, an athlete or a beginner, everyone can benefit from incorporating flexibility and mobility exercises into their routine. Let's explore how you can do these exercises at home and why they're so important.

Flexibility exercises involve stretching your muscles to improve your range of motion. When your muscles are flexible, you can move more freely and easily. Mobility exercises, on the other hand, focus on moving your joints through their full range of motion. Together, these exercises can help you perform daily activities more easily and with less pain.

Start with a gentle warm-up to prepare your body for stretching. Spend five to ten minutes doing light activities like walking in place, arm circles, or gentle marching. This increases blood flow to your muscles and makes them more pliable, reducing the risk of injury.

One of the most basic and effective flexibility exercises is the forward bend. Stand with your feet hip-width apart. Slowly bend forward at the hips, reaching towards your toes. Keep your knees slightly bent if needed to avoid straining your lower back. Hold the stretch for 15 to 30 seconds, feeling the stretch in your hamstrings and lower back. This exercise helps to improve the flexibility of your back and legs.

Another great stretch is the seated hamstring stretch. Sit on the floor with one leg extended and the other leg bent, with the sole of your foot resting against your inner thigh. Reach towards your toes on the extended leg, keeping your back straight. Hold the stretch for 15 to 30 seconds, then switch legs. This stretch targets your hamstrings, which can become tight from sitting for long periods.

For your upper body, try the shoulder stretch. Stand or sit comfortably. Reach one arm across your chest, using your other arm to gently pull it closer to your body. Hold the stretch for 15 to 30 seconds, feeling the stretch in your shoulder and upper back. Switch arms and repeat. This stretch helps to relieve tension in your shoulders and improve your shoulder mobility.

The cat-cow stretch is excellent for improving flexibility in your spine. Start on your hands and knees in a tabletop position. Inhale and arch your back, dropping your belly towards the floor and lifting your head (this is the cow position). Exhale and round your spine, tucking your chin towards your chest and pulling your belly button towards your spine (this is the cat position). Move smoothly between these two positions for 30 seconds to a minute. This exercise increases the flexibility of your spine and can help relieve back pain.

For your hips, try the butterfly stretch. Sit on the floor with the soles of your feet pressed together and your knees bent out to the sides. Hold your feet with your hands and gently press your knees towards the floor with your elbows. Hold the stretch for 15 to 30 seconds, feeling the stretch in your inner thighs and hips. This exercise helps to open up your hips and improve their flexibility.

Now, let's move on to some mobility exercises. These exercises help to improve the range of motion in your joints and keep them functioning well.

One simple and effective mobility exercise is the hip circle. Stand with your feet hip-width apart and place your hands on your hips. Make circles with your hips, moving them in a clockwise direction for 15 seconds, then switch to counterclockwise for another 15 seconds. This exercise helps to loosen up your hip joints and improve their mobility.

Ankle circles are great for improving the mobility of your ankles, which is important for balance and stability. Sit or stand with one leg lifted slightly off the ground. Rotate your ankle in a circular motion, first clockwise for 15 seconds, then counterclockwise for another 15 seconds. Switch to the other ankle and repeat.

This exercise helps to prevent stiffness and improve the range of motion in your ankles.

The wrist stretch is useful for improving wrist flexibility and mobility, especially if you spend a lot of time typing or using your hands. Extend one arm in front of you with your palm facing up. Use your other hand to gently pull your fingers back towards your body, stretching your wrist and forearm. Hold for 15 to 30 seconds, then switch arms. This stretch helps to relieve tension and improve flexibility in your wrists.

Shoulder rolls are excellent for maintaining the mobility of your shoulder joints. Stand or sit with your arms relaxed at your sides. Slowly roll your shoulders forward in a circular motion for 15 seconds, then roll them backward for another 15 seconds. This exercise helps to release tension and improve the range of motion in your shoulders.

The spinal twist is a fantastic mobility exercise for your back. Sit on the floor with your legs extended. Bend one knee and place your foot on the outside of your opposite thigh. Twist your torso towards the bent knee, using your opposite arm to press against your knee for a deeper stretch. Hold for 15 to 30 seconds, then switch sides. This exercise helps to improve the mobility of your spine and can relieve lower back tension.

Don't forget about your neck. Gentle neck stretches can improve flexibility and reduce stiffness. Sit or stand with your back straight. Slowly tilt your head to one side, bringing your ear towards your shoulder. Hold for 15 to 30 seconds, then switch sides. Next, tilt your head forward, bringing your chin towards your chest, and hold for another 15 to 30 seconds. These stretches help to release tension and improve the flexibility of your neck muscles.

Yoga is an excellent way to combine flexibility and mobility exercises. Poses like Downward Dog, Child's Pose, and Warrior II stretch multiple muscle groups and improve joint mobility. You can follow along with online yoga classes or create your own routine. Yoga not only enhances flexibility and mobility but also promotes relaxation and mental well-being.

Incorporating flexibility and mobility exercises into your daily routine can make a big difference in how you feel and move. Aim to do these exercises at least three to four times a week. You can do them as a standalone session or as part of your warm-up or cool-down.

Pay attention to your body and avoid pushing yourself too hard. Stretch until you feel a gentle pull, but not pain. With regular practice, you'll gradually see improvements in your flexibility and mobility.

Flexibility and mobility exercises are a key part of a balanced fitness routine. They help to keep your muscles and joints healthy, improve your range of motion, and reduce the risk of injury. By incorporating these exercises into your routine, you'll be able to move more freely and comfortably, making everyday activities easier and more enjoyable.

Flexibility and mobility exercises are essential for maintaining a healthy, well-functioning body. Start with a gentle warm-up, then incorporate stretches and mobility exercises for different muscle groups and joints. Include yoga for a comprehensive approach, and remember to practice regularly. With consistent effort, you'll see improvements in your flexibility, mobility, and overall well-being.

Chapter 17: Tracking Your Progress

Tracking your progress is a crucial part of any fitness journey. It helps you see how far you've come, stay motivated, and make necessary adjustments to reach your goals. Whether you're new to working out or a seasoned fitness enthusiast, keeping track of your progress can make your workouts more effective and rewarding. Here's how to do it effectively.

Start by setting clear, achievable goals. Decide what you want to achieve, whether it's losing weight, gaining muscle, improving endurance, or just feeling healthier. Having specific goals will give you something concrete to work towards and help you stay focused. Write down your goals and keep them in a place where you can see them often. This will remind you of your purpose and keep you motivated.

Once you have your goals, choose the right tools to track your progress. A simple method is to keep a workout journal. In this journal, write down each workout you do, including the exercises, sets, reps, and weights used. Also, note how you felt during and after the workout. This will help you see patterns and understand what works best for you. If you prefer digital tools, many fitness apps are available that can track your workouts, nutrition, and progress over time.

Another important aspect to track is your measurements. Regularly measuring your body can help you see physical changes that might not be obvious from the mirror alone. Use a tape measure to record the size of key areas like your waist, hips, chest, arms, and legs. Take these measurements once a month to monitor changes. Keep in mind that muscle gain and fat loss might not always show immediate changes on the scale, but measurements can give you a clearer picture.

Recording your weight is another common way to track progress, especially if weight loss or gain is one of your goals. Weigh yourself at the same time each day or week to get consistent results. Remember, weight can fluctuate due to various factors like water retention, so don't get discouraged by minor changes. Focus on long-term trends rather than daily fluctuations.

Tracking your workout performance is also crucial. Note improvements in the number of reps, sets, or the amount of weight lifted. If you're running or cycling, keep track of your distance, speed, and time. Seeing these improvements can be incredibly motivating and show that your hard work is paying off.

Another useful way to track progress is by noting how you feel. Keep track of your energy levels, mood, and any physical changes or improvements. If you notice that you're feeling more energetic, sleeping better, or experiencing less stress, it's a sign that your fitness routine is having a positive impact on your overall well-being.

Photos can also be a powerful tool for tracking progress. Take regular photos of yourself from different angles in the same lighting and clothing. Comparing these photos over time can help you see changes that might not be noticeable in the mirror. Make sure to take these photos consistently, such as once a month, to get the most accurate picture of your progress.

Review your progress regularly to stay on track. Set aside time each week or month to look back at your journal, measurements, and photos. This review helps you see how close you are to reaching your goals and allows you to make any necessary adjustments to your fitness plan. If you're not seeing the progress you expected, consider modifying your workouts, adjusting your diet, or seeking advice from a fitness professional.

Celebrate your achievements, no matter how small. Recognizing your progress and rewarding yourself can keep you motivated and make your fitness journey more enjoyable. Rewards can be simple, like treating yourself to a relaxing bath, enjoying a favorite healthy snack, or buying new workout gear.

Remember that progress isn't always linear. There will be ups and downs along the way, and that's perfectly normal. Be patient with yourself and keep a positive mindset. Consistency is key, and even when progress seems slow, every effort you make brings you closer to your goals.

Tracking your progress is not just about recording numbers; it's about understanding your journey and celebrating your successes. By keeping a detailed record, setting clear goals, and regularly reviewing your progress, you'll stay motivated and on track. This approach will help you achieve your fitness goals and maintain a healthy, balanced lifestyle.

Tracking your progress is an essential part of reaching your fitness goals. Use tools like a workout journal, measurements, weight records, and photos to monitor your journey. Regular reviews and celebrations of your achievements will keep you motivated and focused. Remember, progress takes time, so be patient and stay consistent. With dedication and the right tools, you'll see the results of your hard work and enjoy the benefits of a healthier, stronger you.

Chapter 18: Staying Motivated

Staying motivated can be one of the biggest challenges when it comes to maintaining a fitness routine. It's easy to start strong, but keeping up the enthusiasm over the long haul requires some extra effort. However, with the right strategies and mindset, you can keep your motivation high and reach your fitness goals. Here's how to stay inspired and committed to your fitness journey.

First, it's important to set clear and achievable goals. Goals give you something concrete to work towards and help you measure your progress. Start with small, short-term goals that are easily attainable, like exercising three times a week or increasing your running distance by a small amount. As you achieve these smaller goals, you'll build confidence and feel more motivated to tackle bigger challenges.

Celebrate your successes, no matter how small. Every time you reach a goal or make progress, take a moment to recognize and reward yourself. Celebrations can be simple, like enjoying a healthy treat, taking a relaxing bath, or buying new workout gear. Celebrating your achievements keeps you motivated and reminds you that your efforts are paying off.

Another way to stay motivated is to find an exercise routine that you enjoy. It's much easier to stay committed to something you look forward to. Try different activities to see what you like best—whether it's dancing, hiking, swimming, or yoga. When exercise is fun, it won't feel like a chore, and you'll be more likely to stick with it.

Variety is key to keeping your workouts interesting. Doing the same routine over and over can become boring and lead to a lack of motivation. Mix things up by trying new exercises, changing your workout format, or exploring different fitness classes. Variety keeps your workouts fresh and exciting and helps you stay engaged.

Having a workout buddy can also boost your motivation. Exercising with a friend or family member makes the experience more enjoyable and provides accountability. You're less likely to skip a workout if someone else is counting on you. Plus, sharing your fitness journey with someone else can make the process more fun and rewarding.

Setting a routine helps make exercise a habit. Try to work out at the same time each day or week to build consistency. When exercise becomes a regular part of your schedule, it's easier to stick with it. Make it a non-negotiable part of your day, just like eating or sleeping.

Track your progress regularly to stay motivated. Seeing how far you've come can be incredibly encouraging. Keep a workout journal or use a fitness app to record your achievements. Tracking your progress allows you to see the results of your hard work and reminds you that you're moving closer to your goals.

Staying motivated also involves overcoming obstacles. There will be days when you feel tired, busy, or simply not in the mood to work out. On those days, remind yourself of why you started and the benefits of sticking with your routine. Sometimes just getting started is the hardest part, and once you're in motion, it's easier to keep going.

Make your workouts more enjoyable by incorporating activities you love. Listen to your favorite music, watch an entertaining TV show, or use workout videos that you find motivating. Creating a positive and enjoyable workout environment can help make exercising something you look forward to.

Creating a vision board can be a powerful motivational tool. Visualize your goals and the results you want to achieve by creating a board with images and phrases that inspire you. Place it somewhere you can see it daily to remind yourself of your goals and keep your motivation high.

Another technique is to remind yourself of the benefits of exercise. Whether it's improved health, increased energy, better sleep, or a boost in mood, focusing on the positive effects of working out can help you stay motivated. Keep a list of these benefits handy so you can refer to them whenever you need a motivational boost.

Joining a fitness community, either online or in person, can provide additional support and encouragement. Connecting with others who share your fitness goals can offer motivation, advice, and a sense of camaraderie. Participate in online forums, social media groups, or local fitness events to stay engaged with a supportive community.

Lastly, be kind to yourself. Everyone has off days, and it's important not to be too hard on yourself if you miss a workout or don't meet a goal right away. Treat yourself with compassion and use any setbacks as learning experiences. Remember that progress is a journey, and every step you take, no matter how small, brings you closer to your goals.

Staying motivated requires a combination of clear goals, regular celebrations, enjoyable activities, and consistent routines. Find what works for you, track your progress, and don't be afraid to mix things up. Seek support from others and remind yourself of the benefits of exercise. Most importantly, be patient and kind to yourself. With these strategies, you can keep your motivation high and continue making progress toward your fitness goals.

Chapter 19: Overcoming Common Challenges

Starting and maintaining a home gym routine can be exciting, but it also comes with its own set of challenges. Knowing how to overcome these challenges can make your fitness journey smoother and more enjoyable. Here are some common obstacles you might face and practical ways to tackle them.

One of the biggest challenges is finding time to work out. With busy schedules, it's easy to let exercise fall by the wayside. The key is to make fitness a priority. Schedule your workouts just like any other important appointment. Find a time that works best for you, whether it's early in the morning, during lunch breaks, or in the evening. Even short workouts are better than none. Consistency is more important than the length of each session.

Another common challenge is staying motivated. It's normal to feel excited at first and then see your enthusiasm wane. To keep your motivation high, set clear, achievable goals and track your progress. Celebrate your successes, no matter how small. Remember why you started and the benefits you're working towards. Finding a workout buddy or joining an online fitness community can also provide support and encouragement.

Limited space can be an issue, especially if you don't have a dedicated room for your home gym. Get creative with the space you have. Use multi-functional furniture, such as a foldable bench or stackable weights, to save space. You can also use bodyweight exercises that don't require much room, like push-ups, squats, and lunges. If possible, use outdoor spaces for some of your workouts to get fresh air and more room to move.

Equipment costs can be a barrier for many people. You don't need to buy everything at once. Start with the essentials, like resistance bands, a yoga mat, and a few free weights. Look for second-hand equipment or sales to save money. Over time, you can add more equipment as your budget allows. You can also make your own equipment with items you have at home, like using water bottles as weights or a chair for step-ups.

Another challenge is knowing what exercises to do. With so much information available, it can be overwhelming. Start with a simple, balanced routine that includes cardio, strength training, and flexibility exercises. Many online resources offer free workout plans and videos. Consider following a structured program that fits your fitness level and goals. If you're unsure, consulting a fitness professional for guidance can be very helpful.

It's also common to face physical challenges, such as injuries or chronic pain. It's important to listen to your body and not push through pain. Modify exercises to suit your abilities and avoid movements that cause discomfort. Focus on low-impact activities, like swimming or cycling, which are gentler on your joints. If you have a medical condition, consult with your doctor or a physical therapist before starting a new exercise program.

Mental barriers, such as lack of confidence or fear of failure, can also hold you back. Remember that everyone starts somewhere, and it's okay to be a beginner. Focus on your progress, not perfection. Break your goals into smaller, manageable steps, and celebrate each achievement. Surround yourself with positive influences, whether it's friends, family, or an online support group. Building a positive mindset can make a big difference in overcoming mental obstacles.

Another challenge is staying consistent. Life can be unpredictable, and it's easy to let exercise slide when things get busy. Create a routine that fits your lifestyle and be flexible with it. If you miss a workout, don't get discouraged—just get back on track as soon as you can. Consistency is key to seeing results, so make exercise a regular part of your life.

Balancing exercise with other responsibilities can be tough. Prioritize your time and look for opportunities to incorporate physical activity into your daily routine. Take short walks during breaks, do quick workouts while watching TV, or involve your family in active play. Finding ways to stay active throughout the day can help you stay on track even when life gets busy.

Nutrition is another important factor in your fitness journey. Eating a balanced diet can fuel your workouts and help you recover. Plan your meals and snacks to support your fitness goals. Stay hydrated and focus on whole foods like fruits, vegetables, lean proteins, and whole grains. Avoid processed foods and sugary drinks that can undermine your efforts.

Rest and recovery are often overlooked but are crucial for progress. Make sure to get enough sleep and take rest days to allow your body to heal and grow stronger. Overtraining can lead to burnout and injuries, so listen to your body and give it the rest it needs. Incorporate activities like stretching, yoga, or foam rolling to aid in recovery.

Overcoming common challenges in your home gym journey involves a combination of planning, flexibility, and persistence. Make time for workouts, stay motivated, and get creative with your space and equipment. Focus on a balanced routine, listen to your body, and seek support when needed. By tackling these challenges head-on, you can stay on track and enjoy the benefits of a healthy and active lifestyle. Remember, every step you take brings you closer to your fitness goals. Keep pushing forward, and don't give up. Your effort and determination will pay off.

Chapter 20: Expanding and Updating Your Home Gym

As you progress in your fitness journey, you might find that your home gym needs some updates or expansions. Whether you're looking to add new equipment, make better use of your space, or simply freshen things up, expanding and updating your home gym can keep your workouts exciting and effective. Here's how to do it in a way that's practical and enjoyable.

First, take a good look at your current setup. Assess what's working well and what could be improved. Are there pieces of equipment you rarely use? Are there any areas that feel cramped or cluttered? Understanding what you have and what you need is the first step in making smart updates. Write down your thoughts and ideas so you can plan effectively.

How to make a home gym

Start by thinking about your fitness goals. Have they changed since you first set up your home gym? Maybe you've become more interested in strength training, or perhaps you want to focus more on flexibility and mobility. Your goals will guide your decisions on what equipment and changes are necessary. For example, if you're aiming to build more muscle, adding a squat rack or adjustable dumbbells might be a good idea.

Next, consider the space you have available. If you're working with a small area, think about ways to maximize it. Wall-mounted racks can save floor space, and foldable equipment can be stored easily when not in use. If you have the option, consider moving your gym to a larger room or even using part of your garage or basement. More space means more possibilities for diverse workouts.

Adding new equipment can breathe new life into your home gym. Look for versatile pieces that can be used for multiple exercises. For instance, a set of resistance bands can be used for strength training,stretching, and even some cardio exercises. An adjustable bench can be used for a variety of weightlifting exercises and can also serve as a platform for step-ups and other movements.

Think about the types of workouts you enjoy and how you can enhance them. If you love cardio, a treadmill, stationary bike, or rowing machine could be a great addition. For strength training enthusiasts, consider adding a power rack, barbells, and more weight plates. If flexibility and mobility are your focus, yoga mats, foam rollers, and balance balls can be very useful.

Don't forget about technology. There are many apps and devices that can enhance your workout experience. Fitness trackers can monitor your progress, heart rate, and calories burned. Smart mirrors and interactive fitness screens can provide guided workouts and feedback, making your home gym feel more like a professional studio. These tech additions can keep you motivated and help you stay on track with your goals.

Creating a comfortable and motivating environment is also important. Freshen up the space with a new coat of paint or some motivational posters. Good lighting can make a big difference, so make sure your gym is well-lit. If possible, set up near a window to let in natural light. Adding some plants can also make the space feel more inviting and help with air quality.

Updating your flooring can improve both the safety and comfort of your home gym. Rubber mats or foam tiles provide a cushioned surface that's easy on your joints and protects your floors from heavy equipment. These materials are also easy to clean and maintain. If you're into high-impact activities like jumping or running, a shock-absorbing floor can make your workouts more comfortable and reduce the risk of injury.

Another important aspect of updating your home gym is organization. A cluttered space can be distracting and unsafe. Use storage solutions like shelves, hooks, and bins to keep your equipment neatly arranged. Labeling your storage areas can make it easier to find what you need quickly. A tidy gym not only looks better but also makes it easier to focus on your workouts.

As you add new equipment and make changes, remember to maintain what you already have. Regularly check your equipment for wear and tear and clean it to keep it in good condition. Keeping your gym well-maintained ensures that it's always ready for a great workout and can extend the life of your equipment.

Lastly, updating your home gym is an ongoing process. Your fitness needs and interests may change over time, so stay flexible and open to making further adjustments. Keep an eye out for new fitness trends and technologies that might enhance your workouts. Regularly reassess your gym to make sure it's meeting your needs and helping you achieve your goals.

Expanding and updating your home gym can keep your workouts fresh and exciting. Assess your current setup, consider your fitness goals, and make practical changes to improve your space. Add versatile equipment, use technology to enhance your experience, and create a comfortable environment. Keep your gym organized and well-maintained, and stay open to making further updates as your needs evolve. By continually improving your home gym, you'll stay motivated and enjoy your fitness journey even more.

Conclusion

Building and keeping a home gym is a great way to improve your health and fitness. From planning your space and budget to choosing the right equipment and designing a motivating workout area, every step helps you create a gym that fits your needs.

In this guide, we've covered how to assess your space, select essential equipment, upgrade to advanced options, and find affordable ways to expand your gym. We've also talked about safety, organization, and maintenance to keep your home gym safe, clean, and effective.

We provided tips on making workout plans, including cardio, strength training, and flexibility exercises. Tracking your progress is important to stay motivated. We also discussed how to overcome common challenges and keep pushing forward.

Remember, fitness is a lifelong journey. Keep learning and adapting as your needs and interests change. Try new exercises, equipment, and resources to keep your workouts exciting. Your home gym shows your commitment to health and fitness. With dedication, you can reach your goals and enjoy the benefits of a healthier, stronger, and more active lifestyle.

Thank you for reading this guide. We hope it gives you the knowledge and motivation to create and enjoy a home gym that supports your fitness journey.

Made in the USA
Monee, IL
14 December 2024